Aiming At Life

TARGETING ICE AGAINST PROSTATE CANCER

by

Stephen Scionti, M.D.

authorHOUSE®

AuthorHouse™
1663 Liberty Drive, Suite 200
Bloomington, IN 47403
www.authorhouse.com
Phone: 1-800-839-8640

First published by AuthorHouse   7/17/2008

ISBN: 978-1-4343-6266-7 (sc)

Library of Congress Control Number: 2008900932

Printed in the United States of America
Bloomington, Indiana

This book is printed on acid-free paper.

To The Reader: This book is not medical advice, nor intended to substitute for such. It is not the author's intent to give medical advice contrary to that of an attending physician. For questions of a personal medical nature, please consult your physician.

Cryocare Center
Coastal Carolina Urology Group, LLC
8 Hospital Center Blvd., Suite 150
Hilton Head Island, SC 29926
1-866-422-2284

CONTENTS

ACKNOWLEDGMENT

I am grateful to Endocare, Inc. for the consultation they provided on the technology of CryoCare® as well as permission to use their illustrations. I also want to thank their consultant, Karen Barrie, M.S. for her support and suggestions in making this book as user-friendly as possible.

Introduction

MY PASSION, AND FOUR QUESTIONS

The things I care most about as a doctor had their roots in my childhood. I grew up in Waterbury, Connecticut, the oldest of five kids. My grandparents were Italian immigrants, and a close-knit clan surrounded me. I saw my grandparents every day. Sundays brought the big afternoon dinner with cousins, aunts and uncles. Our family was amazingly healthy. We had the usual cases of childhood ailments but I can hardly remember seeing a doctor. If anything, we probably took good health for granted. Since I didn't have what you might call a medical role model while growing up, my professional ideals stem from universal family values. My parents and relatives embodied a love of family coupled with hard work. There was an atmosphere of expectation, of achieving high standards. I was raised to believe that an education was the most important thing you could get. All of this had a profound effect on how I practice medicine. I try to educate patients about what's going on in their bodies and what we can do about it. I take a teamwork approach to problem solving. I work hard to help patients feel they are receiving the best therapies available. I expect the entire experience of diagnosis, decision, treatment and recovery to enfold them in a cocoon of excellent care. I strive for the highest level of personalized service. In short, I try to treat my patients as I would my own family.

When I finished medical school and completed my residency, I had the zeal of youth. I believed I could be an expert at everything! Experience taught me otherwise, and with it came the wisdom of narrowing my focus. I learned to figure out what I was really good at, and to improve on how it was already being done. I came to believe that I could provide a much higher level of expertise by concentrating on specific diseases.

I developed a particular interest in prostate cancer. There is such a wide range of treatment options that each patient requires complete and careful diagnosis, and enough time to weigh the best possible treatment approach. We know there are different lines of prostate cancer cells, but no one has been able to do the kind of clinical research needed to know which treatment might work best with each line. In fact, I routinely offer a wide range of diagnostic tests, even at the cellular level, in order to understand each patient's disease fully. Only then can I educate that person about prostate cancer, and together with their close family members we can make an informed decision about their care plan. This is my **first objective** as a doctor. I want my patients to see me as their teacher, coach, advisor and partner in their battle against this disease. I welcome the fact that in today's world, with all the latest books and internet resources, many of my patients arm themselves with sophisticated information before we begin, and as we work together.

The history of medicine reveals shifting thoughts and ideas. Today, more and more doctors embrace a mission to the whole person, not just to a body part or a set of symptoms. Likewise you, as a consumer of medical services, are also part of growing awareness that medical practices can affect your quality of life. I am passionate about healing people in a way that not only saves lives, but that also enhances lifestyle. It's a fact that all prostate cancer treatments—let me repeat, ALL—have some possibility, however small, of side effects. Taking the prostate gland out, or destroying it within the body, can affect elimination and sexual performance. Thus, my **second objective** is to combine treatment excellence with an absolute minimum of lifestyle problems.

If I have done a good job with my first two goals, my **third objective** flows naturally. I want each patient to be comfortable with his treatment decision, confident that he has chosen the best solution for the problem, particularly prostate cancer.

Finally, my **fourth objective** is a positive recovery experience. Here in coastal South Carolina I have some unique assistance in achieving this aim. While no geographic place is a perfect paradise, I established my practice where the elements provide a special nurturing that comes from Nature. I know from my own experience how regenerating the relaxing qualities of the ocean can be. All physicians seek access to state-of-the-art, impeccably maintained offices and hospital facilities. I discovered the additional, often intangible, healing benefits of quiet beaches, sweet birdsong, mystical Spanish moss, and fragrant fresh air. I feel very fortunate to have Nature's blessings as part of our "recovery team" along with our professional and very special staff members and nurses.

Now that you know about my philosophy of medicine, and how I see myself, I want to share why I wrote this book about a specific prostate cancer treatment called **cryotherapy**, or the use of lethal ice to treat and destroy cancer in the body. As long as a prostate malignancy has not yet spread to other parts of the body, freezing is a very good option for low, medium, and high risk localized prostate cancer, regardless of the cell line.

The year 2005 was a landmark year for cryo with the publication of long-term (10 year) data on its success. I felt the time was ripe to write a book about it. I have witnessed the success of this treatment, and the high satisfaction of my cryo patients. I am amazed that cryo equipment manufacturers, and the doctors who use it, have not done a better job of getting the word out to patients when the message is so hopeful. It's high time for widespread patient awareness of an exciting "Ice Age!" There is persuasive data that cryo delivers **effective results** as good as, if not better than, traditional therapies, including surgery and radiation, with **minimal side effects.** While I use cryo to treat prostate cancer, it is gaining credibility and popularity for kidney, bone, liver, lung and breast cancers. I expect the list to grow as the news spreads about the advantages of freezing malignant tumors in order to demolish them for good.

Before I began writing, I asked myself four questions:

1) Why would I, a urologist, want to write a book?

2) Why would I want to write it about cryotherapy?

3) What can cryotherapy offer patients whose first-line treatment was radiation but the cancer has come back?

4) Why should readers of this book consider cryo?

I address these questions in the following chapters, but here's a summary of where I'm going with them:

1) Urology is the branch of medicine that deals with prostate cancer treatment and referrals. As a urologist, I review what the prostate gland does, how prostate cancer is diagnosed, and treatment decisions and consequences from a urologist's perspective.

2) Cryotherapy is a first-line approach to curing cancer by administering a lethal freeze to the tumor. I explain the various approaches to treating local prostate cancer, and reveal the advantages of cryo from a patient's viewpoint.

3) Cryotherapy is also a "salvage" approach with the potential to cure cancer if radiation therapy fails and localized prostate cancer has recurred or come back. I devote a separate chapter to explain when salvage cryo may be appropriate, and why it has a competitive edge over other salvage methods.

4) If you have prostate cancer you, not your doctor, have to live daily with the outcome of treatment. There is not one right treatment for everyone. I review key points to help you evaluate if the benefits of cryo ring true for you.

By the time you finish this book, you will be in a position to have an informed discussion with your physician about cryo, if he or she has not already brought it to your attention. I hope that you will agree with me that ice offers distinct advantages. Cryotherapy saves **both life and lifestyle,** as you are about to learn.

Chapter 1.

A UROLOGIST COULD WRITE A BOOK...

The homes in the neighborhood where I grew up were all pretty close together. I was a Baby Boomer, and we didn't have computer and video games back then. There weren't organized after-school programs. We had the kids on the block, and left to our own devices all we needed to keep ourselves busy was getting together in one place. It seems wherever we found a piece of grass or a stretch of concrete, we played stickball, basketball or other games. Each of us brought our own abilities and personality quirks. We had a good time because we cooperated well together. If someone's quirk got out line, friendship and harmony usually prevailed. Once in a great while, though, a well-placed intervention was needed to restore order.

Like kids in the neighborhood, the urinary and sexual organs cradled in and around the low pelvic region cooperate well. Each has its own abilities and quirks. The kidneys, bladder and urethra handle urinary filtration and elimination so well that normal urine is free from bacteria, viruses and fungi. The prostate gland and seminal vesicles contribute to sexual function as they produce semen and other fluids during ejaculation. The neurovascular (nerve and vein) bundles that adjoin the prostate promote sexual and emotional pleasure through penile erections. The penis is the male external organ that has both a urinary and sexual function. When all these organs are left to their own devices, most of the time they keep themselves busy, with positive results. But with aging or disease they have quirks that can get out of line. Then the neighborhood needs intervention.

Urologists are physicians who have special interest, training and experience in **genitourinary** malfunction (genital + urinary = genitourinary). If you ask a urologist why he or she decided to specialize in this field, most will answer that urology offers a satisfying blend of medicine and surgery. In other words, we treat disorders of the urinary and sexual systems through a range of interventions including office visits and sometimes operating room visits. If the urological neighborhood and the internal systems connected with it are disturbed by out-of-line quirks, chances are you will be referred to a urologist for evaluation, diagnosis and treatment.

Cryotherapy (also called cryosurgery or cryoablation) is a highly effective treatment for prostate cancer that is also kind to its neighbors. An expert cryosurgeon who performs this minimally invasive treatment can deliver cancer control as good as, if not better than, traditional therapies, and with a low risk of irreversible side effects. If you have prostate cancer or you are at risk of this disease, it is important for you to know what cryo is and what's so good about it. I will guide you step by step. You will learn about the prostate gland, about prostate cancer itself, and the benefits and risks of each treatment option. I hope to convey my absolute conviction that cryo is a great treatment, based on my experience as a physician, and the positive experience my patients tell me they've had. I hope you will come to believe, as I do, that patients with localized prostate cancer should consider cryo as an option, especially when done by an expert.

Prostate cancer is a genitourinary disease. When a routine blood test reveals an elevation in PSA—more on that later—or a digital rectal exam detects an irregularity on the prostate gland, the patient is usually referred to a **urologist** for further tests. The urologist is the **entry point** into the prostate cancer diagnosis and treatment system. Delivering a diagnosis of prostate cancer after a biopsy is not a happy part of our job. If detected early, however, prostate cancer is among the most curable of all malignancies. You may have heard the saying, "A man is more likely to die *with* prostate cancer, not *from* it," and this is true. About 230,000 men in the U.S. will be diagnosed this year. Because we're finding it earlier, and because treatments are getting better at defeating a tumor without destroying a man's quality of life, more men are undergoing minimally invasive treatments that offer high success rates with fewer side effects. There's a new generation of curative approaches, and cryo is a fabulous member of that generation!

Before I get into the details of the prostate gland, let me share a couple of true stories. I have changed the names of the patients, but their case histories are real.

CASE NUMBER I: CHUCK L.

Chuck was 57 when his internist detected an unusually high PSA of 25.7 during a thorough physical. Chuck was shocked when his doctor told him he suspected prostate cancer. Chuck was referred to me for a needle biopsy. Before doing the biopsy, I went over all his lab findings and did a repeat digital rectal exam. I suspected his internist was right, and I was especially concerned because Chuck had a medical history of heart disease (he had bypass surgery at age 38, and had already had a heart attack). The biopsy revealed a Gleason grade of 9 (more later on Gleason grade). Together with his high PSA, Chuck's cancer would be defined as high-risk.

I scheduled a consultation with Chuck and his wife. I always allow at least an hour, as these are very important and intimate meetings. Together, we ruled out surgical removal because of Chuck's cardiac history and because he had a high probability that the cancer had already penetrated the prostate margin. He did not like the idea of radiation, especially since the dose needed for the best chance of cure would be so high that there would be risk of long-term side effects. That left cryotherapy for the best chance of cure, or hormone therapy for long-term cancer management though it's not curative. Since Chuck's life expectancy was more than 10 years, we all felt that going for cure rather than management was the way to go. He and his wife chose cryotherapy.

CASE NUMBER 2: FRANKLIN W.

For a few years before he moved to this area in 2003, Frank's doctor had detected what he described as a ridge on his prostate, but since his PSA had always been low, the doctor wasn't worried. However, when Frank relocated, he wanted a urologist to monitor his situation, and found me. Because I also detected the abnormal mass on his gland, I recommended a biopsy even though his PSA was down to 2.2 from the previous year's 2.9. It turned out that he had a small tumor on the right side with a Gleason of 6.

Again, I asked him and his wife to come in for a three-way consultation. I explained that since he had a low-risk tumor he could expect equal success from all treatments, and went over each of them as well as the possible risks. Frank was not comfortable with surgery or radiation, or the side effects of hormones; since he had a large gland, I explained that he would temporarily need hormones to reduce its size if he wanted either cryo or radiation, since this would make treatment more effective. He seemed most comfortable with the thought of cryo, but wanted to do more research. He went home, and took time to learn all he could on the internet. When he again came to see me, he and his wife had decided on cryo.

LET'S RECAP BOTH CASES

	Age	PSA	Gleason grade	Appropriate Treatment Options	Choice of Treatment
Chuck	57	25.9	9(5 + 4)	Cryotherapy or hormones	Cryotherapy
Franklin	67	2.2	6(3 + 3)	Surgery, radiation, cryotherapy, hormones or a combination of treatments	Cryotherapy

Each of these patients, Chuck and Franklin, had different diagnostic factors when they first came to see me. In the next chapter I will explain these factors in more detail. Both men decided that cryo was the way they wanted their cancer treated. Let's take a look at what they learned about their bodies to understand why cryo was their choice.

The upside of the prostate from Nature's perspective

Only men have a prostate gland. Mother Nature felt it was so important that she tucked it away where it would be well protected. Why is it so important?

1. The **urethra**, or hollow tube that carries urine out of the body, passes directly through the center of the prostate on its way from the **bladder** to the **penis**. Thus, it has a **urinary function**. If the **prostate gland** enlarges, it can squeeze the urethra shut, causing urination to become more frequent, or more difficult. As men age,

the prostate gland tends to grow. A common condition called benign prostatic hyperplasia (BPH) is not life-threatening, but is often the reason why older men get up once or twice during the night to urinate. Also, the larger the gland, the more PSA that's released into the bloodstream. This is also why aging men often experience a gradual upward trend in their PSA blood test, and this normal occurrence is no reason for alarm.

2. The prostate manufactures seminal fluid to keep sperm alive and help move them out of the body during sexual ejaculation (orgasm). The nerves and blood vessels (neurovascular bundles or **NVB**) that make erection possible hug the prostate on either side. Thus the prostate is a vital part of a man's **sexual function**.

This sketch shows how the prostate is located next to larger structures in the pelvic region:

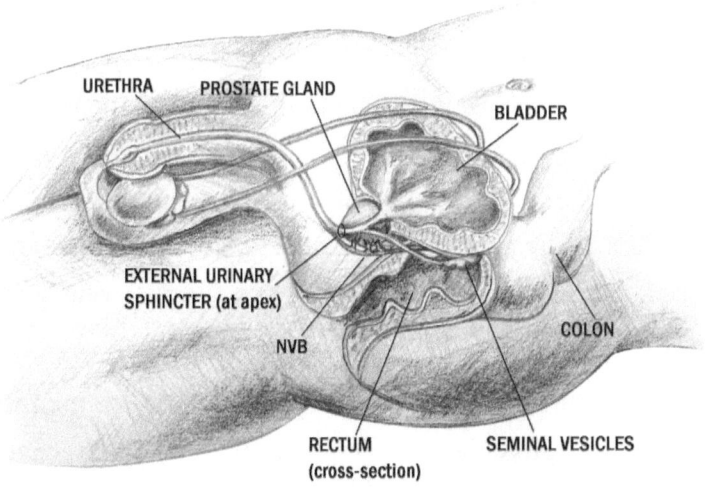

Look closely at how the prostate snuggles up against the bladder, and notice the urethra, leading out of the bladder, through the prostate, to the penis. Where it comes out of the prostate opposite the bladder, there is a very small constricting muscle, the **external urinary sphincter**, with which you voluntarily control urine flow. It is located at the tip, or **apex**, of the prostate.

THE DOWNSIDE OF THE PROSTATE FROM NATURE'S PERSPECTIVE

What are the three most important words in real estate? Location, location, location. As the illustration shows, treating prostate cancer is all about location. Nature designed a dense and protective neighborhood that creates a few medical challenges.

If the prostate becomes diseased, you might not know until you have urinary problems. Any enlargement or inflammation can begin to squeeze the urethra shut, making urination more frequent or difficult. There are three general conditions that result in these symptoms: benign prostatic hyperplasia (BPH); an inflammation or infection caused by an irritant or a biological agent; and cancer, the focus of this book.

Efforts to cure prostate cancer by removing or destroying the entire gland while it's still in the body can have an impact on its next-door neighbors. I call this "collateral damage to innocent bystanders." Any physician who administers a local treatment for prostate cancer does his or her best to avoid this, but there are no guarantees. Here are the main risks:

1. The inability to control urine (leakage or **incontinence**) is a possible treatment side effect. The external urinary sphincter can be damaged by surgery, radiation or

freezing so urologists are very, very careful with this area. Many prostate cancer tumors occur at the apex, so for these patients, aggressive treatment may result in temporary or permanent incontinence to some degree. Fortunately, there are many good ways to alleviate this symptom—but all my patients tell me they fear having to wear "diapers" more than they fear erectile risks.

2. The inability to have a spontaneous erection (**impotence**) can result from cutting, radiating or freezing the nerve bundles (NVB). Rest assured that as with incontinence, there is a wide array of excellent ways to overcome impotence whether it occurs as a result of prostate cancer treatment, or for any of the other reasons that can lead to it (aging, diabetes, circulatory problems, etc.)

3. Rectal difficulties such as a hole in the rectal wall (**fistula**) or inflammation from radiation damage (**radiation proctitis**) or increased risk of rectal cancer as a result of exposure to radiation are also possible side effects of treatment.

I'll discuss each of these in a later chapter.

LET'S RECAP

1. A healthy prostate gland facilitates **urinary function.**

2. The prostate gland is an important part of **sexual function.**

3. Nature sheltered this important organ by planting it **deep in the lower pelvic region.**

4. Prostate cancer treatment carries a risk of **incontinence.**

5. Prostate cancer treatment carries a risk of **impotence.**

6. Prostate cancer treatment carries a risk of **rectal damage.**

THE UROLOGY VIEWPOINT

Diagnosing prostate cancer is almost always done by urologists. Urologists also treat incontinence and erectile dysfunction, which can occur for many reasons including side effects of prostate cancer therapies. In the U.S., most urologists are first trained as general surgeons and then specialize in urologic surgery and other urology treatment. In other words, we really know genitourinary anatomy and how it connects to the whole body! Put another way, *every* urologist knows enough to write a book about prostate cancer treatment if he or she should choose to do so.

I have a particular interest in prostate cancer because there's such a wide range of treatment options but no clear answer on what an individual patient should do. I have a specific passion about one treatment because I have seen it work so well, and my patients have been so pleased. Patients should be able to understand all the options, and be able to see a urologist who has particular expertise in the option they choose. For beam radiation, the urologist refers his or her patient to a skilled radiation oncologist for such therapy. The trend in medical treatment today is toward minimally invasive therapies. I wanted to become as expert in this disease as possible, and to discover the least invasive, safest and most effective option I could offer my patients in addition to the more traditional approaches of surgery and radiation.

A good urologist should be a skilled surgeon, of course, but there are a few other vital aspects to the job. Compassion is essential, since genitourinary organs are very important, both in terms of physical sensitivity and feelings of privacy and modesty. The ability to teach is very important; patients deserve complete and comprehensible explanations of the problem and available solutions.

In the next chapter I want to give you a quick course on prostate cancer treatment options, their benefits and risks.

Chapter 2.

WHY ICE?

Experience: A good school, but the fees are high.
Heinrich Heine, 19th century German poet/satirist.

Neither my grandfather nor my father went to college, but I learned a lot from the benefits of their hard work. When my mom's father arrived in the U.S. from Naples he was penniless. He realized that survival meant integrating into the culture, and he was very determined to succeed. It was the 1920's, a time when silent movies were just catching on. He got a beginner's job as a movie projectionist. Since he desired good quality of life for him and his growing family, he wasn't willing to settle for a minimal existence. As Hollywood progressed into talkies, he diligently mastered his job and saved his small wages. During the boom years of the Roaring Twenties, he parlayed his way into buying a movie theater. After the 1929 crash of Wall Street, he managed his business well despite the years of Depression, acquiring three more theaters in addition to the first. Everyone in town knew him.

He was an authority in the school of experience. He had paid his dues and earned well-deserved recognition. By the time he was 50 he was able to sell the theaters, retire, and ponder what he would like to do with the rest of his life.

Through my grandfather's example, I learned that when I want to make a case, I must work diligently so its merits earn the recognition they deserve. In the field of medicine, I want to be able to say, "Here's why I think this is a good course to take," and cite the science behind it. I would not be doing you a service if I could not back up my case for cryo as a treatment for cancer if I didn't offer you academic science as well as share what I've learned in the school of experience. In Chapter 1 I gave a short anatomy lesson that is the foundation for discussing what I like about cryotherapy as a treatment for prostate cancer.

In this chapter I wear three different hats. First, I will put my Biology Teacher Hat on to tell you about *cancer cells*. Next, I will don my Physics Teacher Hat to show *how ice kills cancer*. I will then put my Urologist Hat on to describe conventional *localized treatments*: surgical removal (radical prostatectomy); external beam radiation; and radioactive seed implants (brachytherapy). From there, I will explain the procedure of cryotherapy. I have heard patients talk about "the butcher, the baker, the ice cream maker" when they refer to the three most effective approaches to eradicating localized malignant tumors: cutting, burning, and freezing. They mean no disrespect to medicine when they use these terms, but we doctors need to listen to such words, for they often reflect how patients experience our efforts to save their lives. This chapter contains the evidence to show why anyone facing a decision about treatment for localized prostate cancer, regardless of risk level, should seriously consider "the ice cream maker."

THE BIOLOGY OF CANCER CELLS

Ever since I studied cellular biology, I have been astonished over the body's continuous creativity at the microcosmic level. Throughout a lifetime, cells build and are in constant communication with other cells and systems. However, every human being produces many cells that develop abnormally. Cancer begins with cells that have *mutated* or changed spontaneously into selfish brats. When normal cells come into existence, they are programmed to eventually age, stop reproducing themselves and die off. This is called the "cell senescence mechanism." Cancer cells are dangerous because they don't have the same built-in time limitations. They are out of control. Like parasites that use their host for survival, they make clever use of the body's resources. They may be clever, but they're not very smart. In fact, they are on a suicide mission. If left untreated, they eventually destroy their host—which means they die too.

There are many theories about why a cell becomes cancerous or *malignant*, such as aging, viruses, exposure to environmental irritants or toxins, etc. Most of the time abnormal cells have a hard time surviving. They either fail to fit into the body's healthy systems, or the immune system successfully detects and kills them. Sometimes, however, a cancer cell escapes detection by the immune system or is stronger than its defenses. As with all cells, it can reproduce itself and multiply. Cancer cells are *opportunistic* meaning they are like illegal trespassers or squatters who find the first unprotected place where they can settle down, hoping to escape notice. If they cluster into a solid tumor, they take up residence in healthy tissue such as organ, muscle or bone. Like all living cells, they need nutrients and oxygen that are carried in the bloodstream. Did you know that the body can build new blood vessels when needed? Think about a wound that needs blood flow so it can heal—special proteins called *angiogenic growth factors* signal the body to develop new small blood vessels to help heal damaged or diseased tissues. This is normal and healthy, but cancer cells are like sneaky gas thieves who siphon out someone else's tank. They secrete the same proteins in order to create their own exclusive pipeline to bring nutrients and oxygen to fuel the infant tumor's growth. See what I mean by "clever"? It's important that you remember that tumors generate their own blood supply. This process is called *angiogenesis*. Cryo's effectiveness is based not only in killing the tumor cells, but also on destroying their pipeline as well.

Under a microscope, normal cells look well-organized and regular in shape. The more advanced a cancer tumor, the more they look disorganized and chaotic. The appearance of prostate cancer under the microscope is reflected by the Gleason Score. A higher Gleason Score means that the prostate cancer cells are more disorganized, aggressive and faster growing. Gleason Scores higher than 6 reflect higher risk, more active prostate cancer cells. Here's a comparison of normal prostate cells, and moderately aggressive prostate cancer cells:

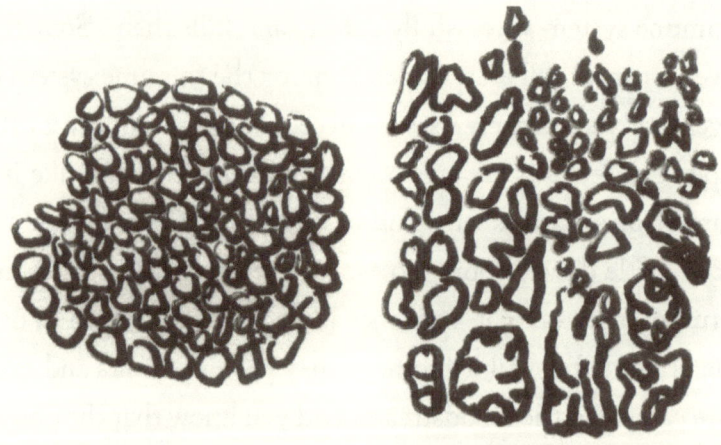

While the tumor is growing, many of its own cells continue to mutate, so what starts as a single cell line begins to produce random adaptations. If a treatment like radiation or chemotherapy is effective against the parent cells, perhaps some of the subsequent mutations may be stronger or more aggressive, capable of resisting treatment. Again, very "clever." If left undetected or unchecked, some cancer cells may spread, or *metastasize*, to other parts of the body. In fact, the tumor's new blood vessels are one way that cells can escape to other part of the body through the bloodstream. From any new location, it can spread again to other locations. If prostate cancer spreads, it is called *systemic disease* because local treatment alone will no longer be effective. Although I will not be discussing treatments for systemic prostate cancer, it is worth noting that with today's hormone and chemotherapy treatments, systemic disease can be well managed for many years.

Prostate cancer treatment therefore has a two-fold objective:

- Remove or destroy the cancer before it spreads and destroys the host (local treatment) or,

- If local treatment is not effective or is too late, maintain control over the systemic disease and manage it like a chronic disease (such as diabetes) to maintain high quality of life for years.

LET'S RECAP

1. Cancer cells are cells that have mutated, or changed, into selfish ones that can destroy their host if undetected and untreated.

2. If they successfully form a tumor, they take advantage of angiogenic growth factors and signal the body to develop their own private blood supply.

3. Cells within a tumor continuously mutate so some may be more resistant to treatments like radiation or chemotherapy.

THE PHYSICS: HOW ICE KILLS CANCER

In college in the '70s, I took both thought-based courses that were like boot camps in logic, and I took science-based courses that were like field training in observation and experimentation. One of my favorites turned out to be biophysics, in which I learned about electrical systems and cell physiology. I had to dissect out the nervous system of a leech under a microscope, and then insert microelectrodes into the nerve cells in order to measure tiny voltage changes. To do so, I had to build some of my own equipment such as oscilloscopes from the type of kits used by electronic hobbyists to build ham radios, etc. There was a good deal of math involved. I came to understand resistance and impedence and the concept of a three-dimensional electronic field. All this college background in logic, math, physics, technology and cellular biology has helped me understand how and why ice is so effective in the treatment of cancer, even though I didn't learn about it until years later when it was well-developed and proven.

Ice is a remarkably adaptable tool. It can even preserve life. Freezing is a great preservative—if you've ever ordered prime steak shipped frozen to your door, or caught a salmon and had it flash-frozen and packed in ice for transport to your own grill, you enjoyed the same great texture and taste as if you cooked it fresh. A technology called *cryopreservation* allows live sperm to be placed in a frozen state for decades with no impact on their viability or fertility. The -196°C temperature is far colder than that used in cryoablation (destruction) of cancer, but a chemical bath enhances the sperm's internal cellular make-up to resist freezing, attaining a state of suspended animation until thawed.

Both extreme cold and extreme heat are lethal to cancer, but the flexibility of ice offers an advantage over heat-based treatments like *radiofrequency* because it preserves structures made of *collagen*. Collagen is a fibrous protein that is abundant in bone, tendons, cartilage, and connective tissue. It is also a component of important body architecture such as the bronchial tubes in the lungs, and in the collecting system of the kidneys. When collagen is exposed to very hot temperatures, it becomes "denatured" and basically turns to gelatin. It cannot return to its original form. On the other hand, it can be frozen and thawed with no significant ill effects. Thus, the preservative nature of ice allows it to be used in and near structures where it would be risky to use a heat-based treatment that could "melt" bronchial tubes or collecting systems. In addition, iceballs have *fixed treatment planes*. This means that the size and shape of the solid ice can be seen with imaging equipment such as ultrasound or CT (computerized tomography), so the physician has a high level of confidence in the exact boundaries of the treated area. Part of the flexibility of ice is its ability to be "sculpted" into the required dimensions.

The same power to preserve cells and tissues can be harnessed equally well to destroy them. Frostbite is an example of harm that, if extreme and prolonged, results in tissue death, or *necrosis*.

However, nature designed cells to withstand exposure to extreme cold, at least for a while. Some creatures, like Antarctic penguins, have adapted to survival at temperatures that would quickly kill us if exposed to them. The use of ice to kill cancer reflects advances in learning how different cells either resist or succumb to freezing.

Success in using extreme cold for curing disease began with treating skin disorders. Over a century ago, physicists discovered how to liquefy gases, producing *cryogens* or agents able to freeze tissue. Dermatologists in the early 20th century found that brief application of liquid nitrogen to external skin conditions such as warts caused their eradication and healing. Sometimes this would occur with only one application, but if the affected area was large or deep, a series of applications was needed for gradual treatment so as not to harm the healthy skin around it. In other words, it is important to limit the zone of destruction <u>only</u> to the necessary area.

After demonstrating for decades how well ice worked on the surface of the body, it was natural to try applying it to internal tumors. In order to explore delivering a lethal freeze to a volume of tissue in a human, scientists faced much clinical research to resolve several unknowns:

1. What happens to cells during freezing?

2. What temperature will guarantee the destruction of all cells?

3. Does the rate of freezing or thawing matter?

4. How long should the freeze be maintained to assure cell death?

5. Does additional damage occur during the thaw?

6. Is there any other damage that occurs afterward?

As the answers emerged, it was found that all these factors interact synergistically, with toxic results for cancer. When properly done, cryo gets rid of cancer as completely as surgical removal.

PHYSICAL CELL DESTRUCTION DURING FREEZING

Killing a cell by freezing it is not as easy as it sounds. Different cells have varying tolerance for extreme cold, and cancer presents a special challenge. Since cells contain water, the formation of ice crystals is a key element in their physical destruction. Water freezes at 0°C*, but mixing it with other chemicals alters the freezing point (e.g. it takes longer to freeze salt water than pure water). The water in cells is such a mixture, contained in the protective cell wall. Fluid also exists in the environment around and between cells, and it begins freezing sooner, so the water inside a cell does not become ice as quickly as the water around it.

When a cryogen is introduced and temperatures start dropping, ice crystals form in the spaces *between* cells, essentially creating a zone of dehydration. The water inside the cells has not yet begun to freeze, and at about -20° an osmosis occurs—water is drawn into the dehydrated zone. The cell now shrinks, which disrupts the protective membrane, and the proteins in the cell are affected in a way that destroys cellular function. Between -20° and -30° most cells will die if the freeze lasts long enough, but in treating cancer nothing is left to chance. Once the temperature falls to -40°, ice crystals now form *within* the cell for the final blow. The stresses on the cell are cumulative: the ice crystals outside the cell wall create abrasive external damage as they form and grow; the internal dehydration created is harmful to cell contents; and the solid formation of internal ice will ultimately destroy the cell from within.

Thus, repeated tests have demonstrated that the *target temperature* of -40° is essential to insure uniform physical cell destruction. Temperatures even colder than that will, of course, kill cancer as well but possibly create unwanted side effects. In cryo, lethal temperature is the most important agent of cell death and easiest to monitor, but other factors also combine for added punch.

TIMING AND OTHER FACTORS

Freezing quickly is more destructive than freezing slowly, but the speed does not seem as important as achieving the target temperature. When a cryoprobe is inserted into a tumor and begins its rapid cooling, tissue closer to the probe freezes sooner than tissue at the edge of the iceball. It is important to give the coldest part of the ice enough time to grow and encompass all tumor cells, so the freeze is maintained for several minutes.

Another crucial element is the process of thawing. As temperatures begin warming toward -20° the ice crystals start to melt and fuse into larger crystals, increasing external pressure on the cell. Water transfers back into it, increasing its volume, and the cell wall ruptures. The cell is now beyond repair. In order to assure no random cell survival, repeating the cycle of freezing and thawing enhances the effect of all processes. Previously frozen tissue is denser and conducts cold for a quicker freeze, with greater uniformity. Any stray survivors now succumb to the repeated forces of the ice crystals, osmosis, chemical concentration and rupture. Therefore, prostate cancer treatment by cryotherapy always involves a *double freeze-thaw cycle*.

Most of the damage I described is complete by the time the dual cycles are done, but further natural breakdown continues during the subsequent days, resulting in complete tumor death. A unique final effect of this treatment occurs within days of cryoablation. Remember when I talked about cancer cells triggering the creation of their own private blood vessels? These small pipelines are referred to as *neovascularity* (*neo* = new, *vascularity* = blood vessels). A very powerful feature of cryoablation is the total destruction of cancer's neovascularity. It begins during the freeze and culminates within several hours of thawing. The freezing process damages the cells that line the blood vessels that supply the tumor. This damage results in thrombosis, or plugging up of the feeding blood vessels. The blood supply to the former tumor is ended, ruling out the possibility of survival. The outcome is the complete and uniform death (*necrosis*) of the tumor. If any "trespassers" had managed to avoid arrest, they would now starve to death.

The iceball produces a sharply demarcated zone of destruction. You may be wondering about the cells at the periphery of the iceball where it touches living tissue at normal body temperature. It stands to reason that the heat of this tissue compromises the target temperature where the iceball's edge comes into contact with it. Because of this, all cryosurgeons add a "margin of safety" and grow the iceball a few millimeters beyond the actual tumor volume. Again, we take no chances of leaving cancer behind, just as a surgeon who is removing a cancerous prostate gland excises (cuts away) as much tissue in the prostate bed surrounding the capsule as he or she safely can. In fact, cryosurgeons can extend the iceball to within 2 – 3 millimeters of the rectal wall. This is a very important advantage in treating aggressive, large tumors that may penetrate the covering or capsule of the prostate and approach the rectal wall.

As I have discussed, ice kills prostate cancer cells in many ways. This becomes especially important in very aggressive, fast growing prostate cancers with Gleason Scores of 7 and higher. These "bad actor" types of cancer cells are particularly resistant to the killing effects of radiation. These cells reproduce quickly and can mutate quickly allowing them to recover from radiation-induced injury. These cells cannot escape as easily from the overlapping deathblows provided by ice.

LET'S RECAP

1. Different cells freeze at different rates, but ice formation is physically destructive as temperatures fall.

2. At -20° ice crystals outside the cell damage its membrane and create a dehydrated state that draws water out of the cell.

3. The internal environment of the cell does not yet freeze but withdrawing water harms cell contents.

4. At -40° ice crystals form within the cell, generating further damage.

5. Since freezing spreads outward from the cryoprobe, maintaining the freeze for several minutes assures that all tissue reaches the uniform target temperature.

6. During the thaw phase, physical destruction occurs as cell membranes rupture.

7. The freeze-thaw cycle is repeated, assuring complete cancer kill.

8. Within hours of the completed treatment, the tumor's blood supply clogs and dies off, eliminating any possibility of cancer survival.

Chapter 3.

CRYOTHERAPY VS. OTHER TREATMENTS

The compelling science of how ice kills cancer and eliminates its blood supply was too good to ignore. Getting precise lethal ice *into* the body without damaging adjacent healthy tissue posed the next challenge. It required real-time ways to "see" the tumor and iceball, to monitor temperature within the iceball as well as at the periphery, and to control the size and shape of the ice.

GETTING LETHAL ICE INTO THE BODY

Back in the '60s and '70s, *visceral* (internal) cryoablation was done by open surgery, since less invasive approaches and imaging were not yet available. Cryosurgeons had to cut the body open to expose the tumor and see where to place the probes and how much ice to generate, though often such surgery exposed only one side or angle of the tumor. Eventually less invasive laparoscopic approaches allowed freezing with minimal surgical openings, but the exact size and shape of the malignancy might not be visible.

It was not possible to monitor temperature, and no one yet knew the correct target temperature or how long to maintain it. Hence, cryosurgeons made educated guesses and froze as aggressively as they dared, but sometimes they created undesirable side effects. Even then they weren't always confident they had encompassed the entire tumor with lethal ice. Since the prostate gland is particularly hard to get to and close to too many other important structures, optimism about prostate cryo dwindled.

In the '90s enthusiasm was renewed by the availability of three advances: sophisticated ultrasound systems; thermosensors that could be placed in and around the site to track temperatures; and cryoprobes that could be inserted directly through the skin under ultrasound guidance. Now cryosurgeons could image the affected organ and tumor from different angles, confirm the exact location of target temperatures, and gain access without open surgery. The original pioneers in prostate cryo included physicians from two different backgrounds. Those with training in radiology (e.g. Duke Bahn, Fred Lee, Gary Onik) were expert at "picturing" internal organs because of their imaging skills with the increasing inventory of tools like ultrasound, CT scans (computerized tomography), MRI (magnetic resonance imaging), etc. Those with training in urologic surgery (e.g. Israel Barken, Doug Chinn, Fletcher Derrick) were expert at pelvic anatomy. Prostate cryotherapy is a natural marriage between the two medical specialties of radiology and urology, and today's technology integrates contributions from both.

Two important lessons began to emerge from the work of these early contributors, including others too many to name:

- If cryo fails to kill all the cancer, rising PSA shows up early, usually within a year, when the most "salvage" treatment options are still open, thus no bridges are burned.

- Most cryo failure is due to undetectable pre-treatment microscopic spread beyond the reach of the lethal ice.

In spite of thorough diagnostic tests like bone scans and imaging of nearby soft tissues and lymph nodes, it is possible to miss early metastasis that has not developed significant mass. In addition to tumor growth into nearby healthy tissue, it can also spread when cells break away into the blood stream via the tumor's angiogenesis, or along nerve lines if the tumor penetrates the tough protective coating that sheathes nerve trunks. Surgical removal "fails" for the same reason—the cancer had undetectably begun to spread.

While this may sound ominous, I am including this information as an indirect proof that ice kills. Surgical removal and cryotherapy both depend on true localization for their success. As long as prostate cancer is contained within the prostate capsule, properly done cryo and properly done surgery have equivalent success. But if the tumor is moderate-to-high risk, enlarging the iceball into a margin of safety beyond the capsule is so powerful at killing cancer that cryo has the best success rates of all treatments, even nosing out surgery and aggressive radiation, when it comes to tumors with a Gleason grade of 7 or higher. Many men who had such high Gleason grades are cancer-free today because their cryosurgeons were able to nip early metastasis in the bud by freezing aggressively.

LET'S RECAP

1. Today's prostate cryosurgery is minimally invasive.

2. There is no open surgery since cryoprobes can be inserted into the gland through the skin.

3. Ultrasound imagery guides probe placement and freezing.

4. Thermosensors in and around the gland monitor real-time temperatures.

5. Since the effects of cryo occur quickly, any recurrence of cancer usually shows up within a year, allowing early decisions about salvage treatment options.

6. If cancer recurs after cryo, it is most often because the cancer had already begun to spread beyond the reach of the iceball.

7. However, the ability to generate a margin of safety often preempts cancer spread, making cryo a highly effective treatment for moderate-to-high risk tumors.

Now let's examine common treatment options: radical prostatectomy (surgical removal), external beam radiation, brachytherapy (implanted radioactive seeds), and combination beam radiation/brachytherapy. I will first briefly describe each treatment and its pros and cons, then return to cryotherapy to see how well it stacks up.

SURGICAL REMOVAL OR RADICAL PROSTATECTOMY

In residency training, urologists are taught that surgical removal of the entire gland is the "gold standard" of prostate cancer treatment. This means that radical prostatectomy, or RP, has the largest and longest statistical track record of all treatment options for prostate cancer. In fact, until external beam radiation was refined, surgical removal was the only way to treat localized prostate cancer. In the 1980's, RP was refined and popularized by Dr. Patrick Walsh at Johns Hopkins. Before the PSA blood test was available, many patients were diagnosed too late for surgery to be curative, resulting in statistical failure rates of 30% or more. Also, it used to be a long operation with risk of too much blood loss, high incidence of post-surgical incontinence, and almost certain impotence. Add in the long recovery, and men over 65 or with certain medical conditions were not considered good candidates for the operation. More accurate diagnosis and new surgical techniques now offer less time under anesthesia, better success, fewer side effects, and shorter recovery.

For an idea of what's involved with removing the prostate, look at this picture:

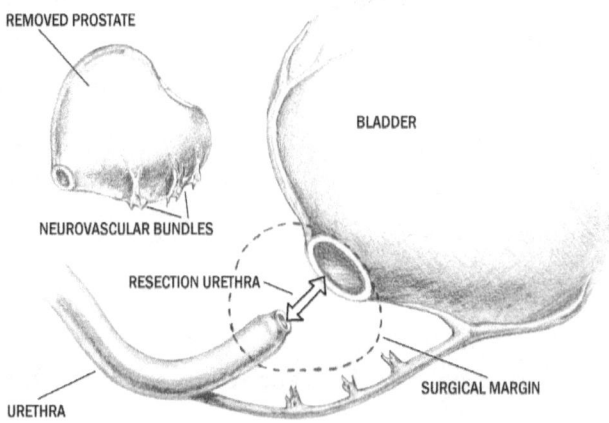

REMOVED PROSTATE

BLADDER

NEUROVASCULAR BUNDLES

RESECTION URETHRA

SURGICAL MARGIN

URETHRA

The gland must be carefully separated away from the bladder and surrounding tissue. The surgeon also removes the seminal vesicles and some of the prostate bed surrounding the prostate. If it is safe to spare the neurovascular bundles on one or both sides, they are gently teased away from the surface of the prostate. Since the urethra passes through the gland, the cut-away end closer to the penis is drawn toward the neck of the bladder and reconnected, and the muscle that controls urination (*external sphincter*) is preserved as carefully as possible. For many patients this part of the surgery, called *resecting the urethra*, results in shorter penile length, but shorter length can be a result of cryo as well.

Radical prostatectomy is still often done as an open abdominal surgery (more invasive), or the surgeon may approach through the perineum, which avoids a large abdominal incision. Today, some urologists are using laparoscopy to access the prostate through several small incisions with special instruments to light, magnify and cut the gland away (laparascopic radical prostatectomy) with shorter and more comfortable recovery. Also, RP can be done with surgeon-guided laparoscopic robotic equipment.

RP always removes the entire prostate.

Depending on how advanced the cancer is, during surgery one or both nerve bundles may also be removed. The nerve bundle can be saved only if there is no cancer near the nerve bundle. Even in the case of a hypothetical tumor with one small focus and no clinical evidence of disease elsewhere, the entire gland will still be removed. Unlike a breast lumpectomy for breast cancer, once the surgeon has gone this far into the body, it would make no sense to leave part of the prostate behind no matter how cancer-free it appeared. No patient would want to go through this surgery twice—or pay double, as RP is a costly inpatient procedure usually followed by 3-5 recovery days in the hospital.

Following surgery, regaining continence may take up to several months; some men never regain full continence, but statistics vary according to the skill of the surgeon and the patient's anatomy. In fact, the success and side effects of RP are "operator dependent," meaning the more experienced the surgeon, the better the results.

If you're considering RP, here are my suggestions:

- Get a highly experienced surgeon (think in terms of at least 150 RP's before yours).

- Ask him about his incontinence rates, and how he defines incontinence (it should be zero pads at any time).

- Ask him how long it typically takes his fully continent patients to get there.

As for potency, it's important to realize that even if your surgeon says he can spare the nerves, he can't give you a 100% guarantee for three reasons:

- Visual observation during surgery may reveal greater cancer progression.

- At time of removal, the gland is immediately sent to an on-site pathologist who inspects it under a microscope. This too may reveal more aggressive disease, necessitating removing one or both nerve bundles.

- Nerve regeneration is unpredictable, so despite a surgeon's best efforts, the trauma of surgery sometimes results in temporary or permanent impairment.

As with all prostate cancer treatments, remember that <u>potency</u> means erectile ability, *not orgasmic ability!* The nerves that control orgasm are separate from those that control erection—you can have an orgasm with or without an erection. Problems with erections can, in most cases, be successfully treated to the satisfaction of a man and his partner.

A prostate cancer patient should consider RP if he is a surgical candidate, if he has low-to-moderate risk disease, and if the thought of surgical removal offers him the greatest psychological comfort. A patient's beliefs and attitude are as important to take into treatment consideration as other clinical and health issues.

LET'S RECAP

Potential benefits of RP include the longest statistical track record of all treatments, more appropriate patient selection thanks to earlier and better diagnosis, less invasive surgery thanks to laparoscopic approaches, the introduction of nerve-sparing surgical techniques, and the psychological reassurance that the cancer is out of the body.

Potential costs of RP include dependence on operator skill and experience, greatest risk of post-treatment incontinence, disappointing loss of potency despite pre-treatment expectations of surgeon, longest recovery of all treatments, risk of shorter penile length, greatest success limited to Gleason grades less than 7.

RADIATION TREATMENTS

Radiation treatment, or radiotherapy, is non- or minimally-invasive, but I call it a blind therapy. We can't accurately see what it's doing while it's doing it. Some people think that radiation kills by generating high heat. This belief is mistaken (e.g. dental X-rays cause no sensation of heat). However, radiation exposure gradually leads to a wound called a radiation burn since it looks and feels like a heat-induced burn. Most normal cells repair radiation damage better than cancer cells. Because of its rapid growth, cancer is more susceptible to radiation and tumor cells can't self-repair as well as normal ones.

There are two approaches to irradiating the prostate gland: external beam radiation therapy (EBRT) 5 days/week over several weeks, or permanent implantation of radioactive seeds into the prostate (*brachytherapy*). Either way, the idea is to bombard the gland with the largest dose of radioactivity "fractionated" over time to give healthy cells the chance to repair themselves during slow exposure. It does not kill cancer quickly, and cancer cells can mutate while the radiation does its job, so long exposure is essential. In prostate cancer treatment, initial incontinence or impotence is rare, and it is effective with low-risk cancers (Gleason < 7). Recall that aggressive, high Gleason Score cancers can mutate and outsmart the radiation treatment.

To understand how it works, think of the cell's genetic duplication code. Radiation corrupts DNA so the cell should become unable to reproduce and eventually die off. It's relatively slow, and can be uneven due to radiation scatter as well as varying cell hardiness. It's impossible to "see" the precise areas of kill, so the key to treatment lies in *dosimetry*, or calculating the most aggressive dose, and focusing it as much as possible. If the tumor proves to be resistant to radiation and cancer returns, repeat radiation is not a future treatment option. Nearby healthy cells can also have their DNA affected, slightly increasing the risk of new cancer onset unrelated to prostate cancer, such as rectal cancer.

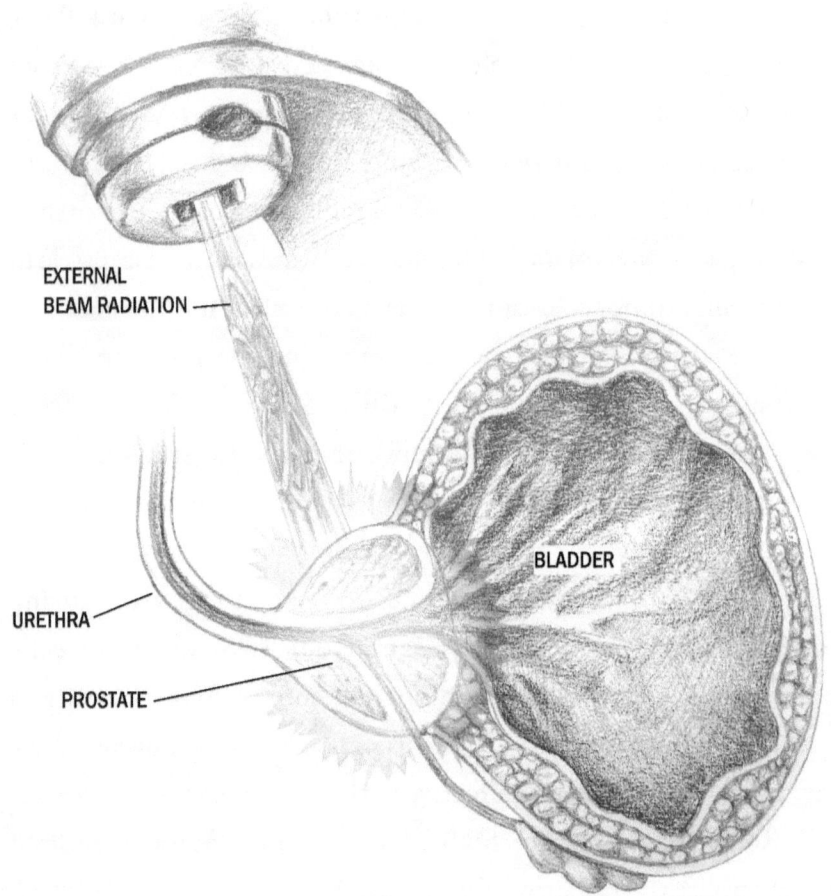

EXTERNAL
BEAM RADIATION

URETHRA

PROSTATE

BLADDER

While there have been improvements, treatment still takes 5-7 weeks. New technologies can target the destructive power more accurately, resulting in more precise kill with less scatter. Side effects such as fatigue, rectal discomfort, diarrhea and urinary symptoms are usually temporary. However, delayed side effects of radiation therapy can emerge even years after treatment. These delayed side effects are due to permanent changes in the neighboring structures, particularly the bladder and the rectum. I think of this as "collateral damage" from the scatter of radiation energy. These delayed problems include: urinary urgency (gotta go), urinary urge incontinence (can't get to the bathroom in time), bleeding from the urinary bladder, rectal urgency, rectal narrowing, and bleeding from the rectum. It is now recognized that erectile dysfunction, or impotence, becomes increasingly common as each year passes after radiation treatment due to long term effects on the neurovascular bundles.

Brachytherapy, or radioactive seeding, is a one-time procedure that permanently implants very small radioactive pellets, or seeds, throughout the prostate tissue under ultrasound guidance. The radiation doesn't pass through the body to target the gland. This procedure has also been improved so there is almost no risk of a seed migrating to other areas of the body, as had occasionally happened previously. The strongest dose of radiation occurs over the first several months, and gradually diminishes. There are usually mild side effects such as frequent urination, urgent urination, burning with urination and occasionally urinary retention or the complete inability to urinate. Patients are cautioned that pregnant women and children not get too close to them for a few weeks, due to risk of radiation exposure. However, long-term side effects may occur years after implantation, since there is no way to protect the bladder, nerve bundles and rectum from radiation scatter. This illustration will give you an idea of seed implants:

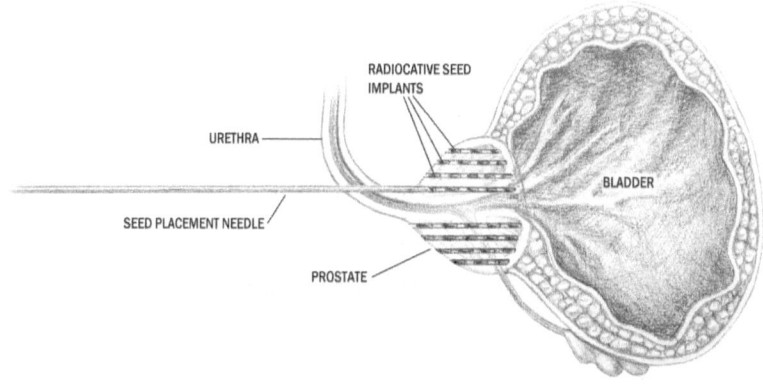

As you will notice, the surgically sharp needle used to implant the seed is similar to the sharp-tipped cryoprobe, and both procedures are minimally invasive since the needles and probes are inserted directly into the gland through the skin, with no incision. A final word about radiation treatments concerns the caregiver. Remember that the urologist is the entry point into prostate cancer diagnosis. If a patient is referred for EBRT, he will then work with a radiation oncologist for the weeks of treatment. Many urologists are now trained to perform brachytherapy, so patients are treated by the same person who diagnosed them. However, in the case of beam radiation, after the treatment is done the patient returns to the urologist for annual PSA follow-up. My professional bias is, the radiologists who offer EBRT rarely see the long-term results of their prostate cancer treatment, so they may not be aware of what we urologists see if post-radiation symptoms appear over the following years. This reinforces my opinion that radiation is a blind treatment, so at least you are aware of my bias.

LET'S RECAP

Potential benefits of radiation include noninvasive (EBRT) to minimally invasive (brachytherapy), appropriate choice for nonsurgical candidates, low rate of immediate side effects such as incontinence and impotence, highly effective for Gleason grade less than 7.

Potential costs of radiation include non-repeatability of radiation to pelvic region even for other cancers such as colon or bladder cancer, need for highest possible dose without side effects, inability to validate by sight the area of cell death, uneven cell death over time, possible survival of hardy cancer cell lines, long-term emergence of post-radiation bowel and erectile problems, and few salvage options if cancer recurs.

Radiation oncologists often see prostate cancer patients for their treatment only, whereas it's the urologists who do the long-term follow-up. Patients do not often have an ongoing relationship with the radiation oncologist who treats them.

CRYOTHERAPY

Turning the prostate gland into a ball of lethal ice with an additional safety margin is a relatively simple procedure. In most cases, it can be done on an outpatient basis if the facility is set up that way. Today's sophisticated, computerized technology makes it possible for an experienced cryosurgeon to complete a straightforward case in about an hour and a half. This means less time under anesthesia for the patient, a savings of time for both patient and physician, and a savings of money since cryo is quite economical compared to RP and radiation.

Here's how it goes. Before cryotherapy, the patient is prepped according to protocol. Then he is given either general anesthesia, or a local with light sedation. A warming catheter is inserted to protect the urethral lining during cryo. An ultrasound probe is placed in the rectum, to "map" the gland size and guide precise placement of probes to maximize ice coverage. When all is ready, the cryosurgeon inserts the slender, surgically-tipped cryoprobes and thermal monitors through the perineum (skin between the scrotum and anus) and confirms their positions before activating the cryogen. Then a double freeze-thaw cycle is implemented, and the physician confirms that target temperatures are reached, and the desired area is encompassed in lethal ice. Here is an artist's image:

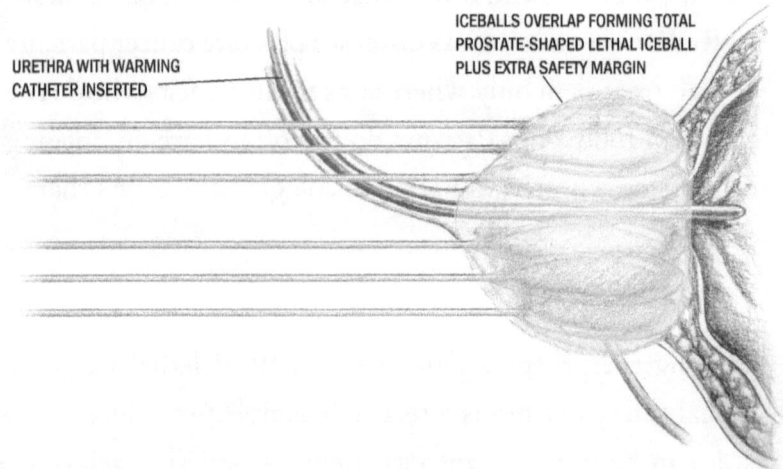

URETHRA WITH WARMING
CATHETER INSERTED

ICEBALLS OVERLAP FORMING TOTAL
PROSTATE-SHAPED LETHAL ICEBALL
PLUS EXTRA SAFETY MARGIN

After the second thaw, the probes, thermal monitors, and ultrasound probe are removed; the warming catheter is generally left in place while the patient is in the recovery room, but will be replaced with a temporary catheter to assist in draining urine during recovery at home. When he is no longer groggy, he is either released, or spends a night at the facility for observation, according to facility protocol and the patient's best interest.

At home, the patient may experience swelling and bruising of the scrotum and surrounding area. Most patients report that any discomfort is manageable with over-the-counter pain medication, but many say they never take anything. Patients are up on their feet and ease back into normal activity within days, and total recovery in most cases, including catheter removal, is 1-2 weeks, with a 2-week restriction against heavy work or exercise. These are normal expectations, but it is not unusual to hear stories of men who made it to their usual bowling night out or shoveled snow off the roof less than a week after cryo. In fact, I recently treated a 52-year old gentleman who completed a 72-hole golf tournament only ten days post-cryo with no ill effects! While I'm not recommending strenuous activity after cryo, he is a perfect illustration of how surprisingly easy most patients say their recovery was.

Urinary incontinence as a side effect of cryo is rare, less than 2%. The majority of men experience 100% continence when the catheter is removed. On the other hand, impotence is a likely side effect of total gland cryotherapy, since the neurovascular bundles are included in the margin of safety. However, a study reported by B. J. Donnelly et al revealed that 47% of patients who had total gland cryotherapy regained full or partial sexual function (some assisted with medication) within 36 months of cryo.[1] And, as with all post-treatment erectile dysfunction, orgasmic ability is not affected by treatment.

Now there are new approaches to preserving potency at the time of cryo, and for encouraging the return of potency in patients who were fully potent prior to cryo. For patients with "unifocal" disease (one tumor focus in one side of the gland, with no clinical evidence of clinically significant tumors elsewhere in the prostate) a partial freeze may be an option. In such a case, an aggressive freeze on the tumorous side of the gland, including the NVB and seminal vesicles on that side, spares the NVB on the non-tumorous side. Early results reported by Dr. Gary Onik (Celebration, FL) and Dr. Duke Bahn (Ventura, CA) indicate about 80% of men are potent following this focal approach to cryo, and over 90% showing no rise in PSA as long as seven years later. *NOTE: these patients are carefully qualified by an intensive "saturation" biopsy, and by their motivation to be scrupulous about frequent follow-up. Since normal prostate tissue is left intact, they will have a normal measurable PSA that is expected, however, to remain stable over time with no indication of rise.*

Another approach to preserve potency is to place a warming probe adjacent to the NVB on one or both sides of the gland. Helium gas, rather than a cryogen, is run through such probes, resulting in protecting the NVB from the freeze. This approach was developed by Dr. David Ellis (Arlington, TX) who feels that all things being equal, any patient who would qualify for a nerve-sparing radical prostatectomy can appropriately be considered for this option.

Finally, even when cryo results in immediate impotence for a man who was potent prior to cryo, recent observation suggests that immediate post-cryo prescribing of medication and/or the use of a vacuum erection device facilitates the regaining of erectile function. More studies need to be done, but the anecdotal evidence is very promising. Remember that nerves are mysterious, and if they are not severed, they may regenerate spontaneously. Helping them along, and meanwhile keeping penile tissue elastic and oxygenated by assisting erectile blood flow into the spongy tissue, appears to facilitate a much quicker return to potency than might have occurred if left to Nature alone.

Now that you know how relatively simple cryo is, with a rapid return to recovery, here is the report of "Chuck" whom I first mentioned in Chapter 1, in his own words:

I went for a thorough physical in November, 2004. Because of genetic factors, I had bypass surgery at age 38, and a heart attack over 10 years ago. My exam included an echocardiogram, treadmill stress test, and colonoscopy. Although I had no prostate or urinary symptoms, I asked for a PSA blood test and digital rectal exam (DRE).

When my internist got all the lab results, he told me, "Your cholesterol is great, your glucose is back to normal, you've lost 3 pounds, and you've got prostate cancer." I was stunned. "Doctor, what did you just say?" My PSA was 25.6, showing not only that I had cancer, but that it was aggressive. I was devastated. "Don't worry," he said, "I made an appointment with a urologist, Dr. Scionti." On the way home, I wondered, "Why is this happening?" When I told my wife and family, we cried about it. It had been easier to deal with my heart problems. To me, the "C" word always had such a final tone to it.

When I met Dr. Scionti for the first time, I found him to be exceptional. He repeated the DRE, and after going over my lab records he agreed with the internist. He ordered an MRI, and scheduled a biopsy around my upcoming camping trip in Georgia. The shots to numb the area were the worst part, but after that I didn't really feel the biopsy sticks. When it was over, Dr. Scionti held my stomach to help ease the sensation of pressure, then he said, "Now if you relax for about five more minutes you can head off to go camping." I drove all the way!

The biopsy revealed a Gleason grade of 9. Dr. Scionti went over each of the treatment options: chemotherapy with radiation; brachytherapy (radioactive seed implants); and cryotherapy. He gave me the full parameters of all three. He did not feel prostate removal was a good option in my case. I knew I did not want chemo, or nuclear medicine, so I decided to go with cryo because it had no chemo or radiation side effects, and could be done outpatient. Meanwhile, he put me on a temporary hormone implant to stop the cancer progression. He assured me, "We're going to take care of you." I said, "I've done my homework and I trust you." It married our openness and respect for each other.

My cryo was scheduled for Wednesday, February 9, 2005. I came in early for the prep, but did not see Dr. Scionti until it was over. To my knowledge the procedure went well. Since I had a suprapubic catheter inserted, the nurses came in and showed me how to wear the leg bag. The following Monday I had the catheter removed by an associate of Dr. Scionti's. Since I hadn't been given a pill to avert bladder spasm, it occurred after the removal. It went away as soon as I got the pill. There were no other bad times in my recovery. I find that amazing.

I saw Dr. Scionti on Tuesday. He apologized and said it never should have happened. By then I was able to urinate with a solid flow and cut-off. However, my penis was shrinking and I had no erection, but Dr. Scionti prescribed use of a vacuum pump. Within a week of regular use, I had full growth and found I could maintain erections. This is personal, a lot of men don't talk about this. Let me just say my wife and I are still at the point of discovery.

When I went to get my PSA checked on my third month anniversary, Dr. Scionti said "There is zero cancer." I know that cryo was the right way to go for me. As for all the emotional issues that go with cancer diagnosis and treatment, the support of my wife and family and my personal faith were very sustaining.[2]

LET'S RECAP

1. Cryotherapy is **minimally invasive** with rapid recovery.

2. Cryo can often be done as an **outpatient procedure** saving time and money.

3. **Incontinence** is a rare side effect of cryo. In fact, cryo has the lowest average incidence of urinary incontinence of all localized treatments.

4. **Impotence** is a common side effect of a total gland freeze, but new approaches to preserving potency for qualified patients show early success of about 80%.

5. **Regaining potency** occurs naturally for almost half of patients at 36 months, but this can be accelerated by immediate post-treatment intervention.

PERSUASIVE STATISTICS

By now I hope I've explained the physics, biology and clinical application of cryotherapy in the fight against prostate cancer. I'm also interested in the statistics reported, the hard and cold data! One of the most persuasive journal articles I read is "A Prospective Trial of Cryosurgical Ablation of the Prostate: Five-Year Results."[3] The average follow-up was 50 months, with biopsies revealing that 72 out of 73 cases were negative for malignancy. For me, this was compelling evidence that cryotherapy is effective. Even longer-term results were published by Dr. Duke Bahn, et al,[4] who reported on 590 consecutive patients with follow-up as far as seven years out from the time of their cryo, evidence of its durable success. These numbers refer to primary cryo, or cryo as a first treatment for localized prostate cancer. In the next chapter I will discuss the use of cryo as a "salvage" treatment for patients who had primary radiation therapy to begin with, but their cancer has come back.

Dr. Bahn's data gave me ample physical evidence of the power of ice as a definitive way to kill cancer. However, in my philosophy, wellness includes not only physical health but also emotional and social well-being. A final study I want to share here was a report on "Quality of Life and Sexuality of Men with Prostate Cancer 3 Years After Cryosurgery," by John W. Robinson, et al.[5] This is an important study because the 75 study participants completed the *Functional Assessment of Cancer Treatment – Prostate (FACT-P)* both prior to their cryotherapy and then afterward at 6 weeks, 3, 6, 12, 24, and 36 months. They also completed a *Sexuality Follow-Up Questionnaire* at three years post-cryo. The categories of well-being that are assessed by the FACT-P are

- physical well-being
- social/family well-being
- emotional well-being
- functional well-being, and
- relationship with doctor.

The authors found that by a year after cryo, all quality of life scales except Social/Family Well-being had returned to pre-treatment levels, and over the next two years remained stable as shown by the results at 36 months. The slightly lower scores on the Social/Family scale seemed attributable to the high rate of impotence following total-gland treatment. However, with the return of erectile function for those who either regained it spontaneously or with medication, the scores rose over time. The other reason this study is valuable is the comparison between post-cryo quality of life with post-treatment with RP, EBRT, brachytherapy and watchful waiting. The authors turned to other published authors to gain this information. Their literature review suggested to them that their sample of cryosurgery patients had higher overall quality of life scores than did those who received the other treatments. This included their relationship with their doctors.

LET'S RECAP

1. Statistics indicate the **high likelihood** of complete cancer kill by lethal freeze.

2. Statistics reveal the **durable, long-term** results of cryo

3. Statistics suggest that after cryo, patients enjoy **generally higher overall quality of life** than patients who receive other treatments.

All of this science confirms my experience: when patients experience little or no pain in their treatment and recovery, when they return to normal life quickly, when they aren't concerned about radiation in their bodies, when they have full bladder and bowel control, when their treatment success is durable, when they see the same urologist who did their treatment year after year for follow-up—all these add up to better whole-person quality of life. I think it accounts for why patients have dubbed cryotherapy "the ice cream maker," a word that sounds kinder than "butcher" or "baker."

To help pay for medical school, I had an experience with an altogether different kind of ice cream maker that saved my education and taught me the value of resourceful persistence, as I had seen in my father and grandfather. I could not have been more grateful to my folks for putting me through prep school and helping pay for college. For my part, I had received some scholarship help and school loans, and had ranked high enough as a junior to be offered a teaching assistantship—the only undergrad at that time to do so. My parents could not have been prouder when their first child graduated with honors from an Ivy League university, but with four kids coming up the line they could offer me no more financial help. If I wanted to go to medical school, I was on my own, with loans to pay off.

After comparing costs, I made the logical and pragmatic choice to relieve the financial pressures. I turned down acceptance at a notable out-of-state program in favor of a room at home and the more affordable tuition at our well-reputed state university. Still, I had to come up with the cash, so I read a little ad in the paper about being a Good Humor ice cream vendor. I thought it sounded very romantic, but it turned out to the one of the hardest things I ever had to do. They said they hadn't had a successful route in my hometown in 10 years, but if I wanted a shot at it, they would rent me the truck at $125 per week, I would buy the ice cream wholesale, and good luck. The hidden costs included running the compressor at night to keep the ice cream frozen, and the rapidly rising fuel costs now that the energy crisis was on. I soon figured out that for inner city kids, ice cream on a hot summer day was an affordable and popular treat. If I was willing to avoid the comfortable but non-lucrative suburban middle-class routes, and truck into the inner city, I could avoid the failures of previous drivers.

So there I was, an Ivy League graduate navigating a Good Humor truck around neighborhoods my peers would have scorned. By dint of determination, tenacity and a dose of street smarts I made enough that summer to pay for my first year of medical school, including tuition, fees, food and even a beater car that I literally paid for with bags of quarters! The following year, the company said I had done so well in town that they would offer me a route on the beach. There was a long shoreline, but competition had discouraged the guy before me, who had not been able to make a go of it. The potential was huge, and my success the previous summer gave me confidence. This time I did even better, thanks to making the acquaintance of a friendly hot-dog vendor I met during the first week of June. He and his girlfriend were very kind and helped me cut expenses as we worked out a mutually beneficial arrangement whereby I paid her a weekly sum to plug my truck into an outlet at her home during the night. If the weather was good, I slept on the beach in a sleeping bag; if not, I slept on top of the freezer in my truck. I took no days off, and worked 12-14 hour days. All the Italian families came to the beach for a week or two of vacation, and when I rang the truck bells, the uncles would come out with a $20 bill and say, "Hey, ice cream for everybody." I started my own business, and I learned to build relationships as each week brought a new crowd. The "ice cream maker" put me through two years of medical school. It also helped me acquire abilities that have turned into lifelong assets.

I found out for myself that persistence, strategic use of resources, and repeated success pay off. The history of the development of cryotherapy is a lesson in how the pioneers of prostate cryo exemplified such qualities. Armed only with the knowledge of how ice physically destroys cells, they persisted in testing target temperatures, duration of freeze, combinations of freezing and thawing, and long follow-up periods to make sure no cancer survived and came back. They strategically utilized new technologies as they became available: thermocouples, smaller probes, imaging methods and computerized algorithms to calculate iceball size and isotherms in order to reduce cryo to a minimally invasive approach. As one success led to another, and word got out to patients who sought out treatment by these pioneers, the number of cryosurgeons grew and the treatment became more refined.

Unfortunately, the same principles that make humans successful also make cancer cells as dangerous as they are. They are persistent in their resistance to self-destruction and tenacious in their mutation. They opportunistically use any avenue of spread, be it nearby tissue, the bloodstream, nerve trunks—whatever. And their repeated success in escaping detection and destruction simply reinforces how out of control they are, until they are the cause of death. This is why it's important to find solid tumors while they are still small, and why a treatment like ice not only encapsulates the tumor but also adds an additional safety margin, to preempt their spread.

I have spent an entire chapter making my best scientific case for why and how lethal ice conclusively destroys any cell subjected to it. This is my world of cryotherapy. It's part of the bedrock philosophy of medicine that guides physicians to offer patients the most caring and effective therapies possible—and above all to do no harm. But we are up against a formidable and resilient foe. Cancer is fierce in its determination to survive. Sometimes, in spite of our best efforts and the best science available, the treatments we prescribe fail. This is why lifelong monitoring of PSA in the bloodstream is essential after prostate cancer treatment, whether RP, radiation or cryo. If the PSA begins to rise, it doesn't always mean the cancer is back, but it is a warning sign that must be heeded!

If PSA is found to rise after radiation therapy, and a biopsy then reveals that prostate cancer is back, cryotherapy occupies a unique position. There is a Medicare-approved back-up strategy called "salvage cryo" for localized recurrence. The next chapter explains why this is such a promising breakthrough.

Chapter 4.

WHEN RADIATION FAILS, ICE COMES TO THE RESCUE

Back when Westerns were popular TV fare, phrases like "circle the wagons" and "hold down the fort" were part of a Baby Boomer's childhood vocabulary. Many programs dramatized tense sieges— setups for the miraculous appearance of reinforcements. "Send in the Cavalry!" was a common battle cry.

When radiation is properly prescribed as a primary (first) treatment—whether beam radiation, seeds, or a combination— one can be confident of successful cancer control. As with other treatments, however, there is never 100% success. Sometimes radiation therapy fails, and reinforcements are needed. On average, 25% of all radiation patients will experience recurrence within less than 5 years. The first sign is usually a *persistent* rise in PSA after treatment—not to be confused with the *temporary bounce* that often occurs after brachytherapy. Note that a rising PSA after radiation or cryotherapy does not necessarily mean recurrence. It may indicate a benign inflammation or infection in the residual prostatic tissue, so it's essential for your doctor to find out where the rising PSA is coming from. On the other hand, an elevated PSA after radical prostatectomy is *always* a warning sign of recurrence, and more diagnostic information is needed to proceed with a treatment plan.

The concept of salvage means saving something already damaged from further destruction or danger. At best, it means rescue of something that was thought to be lost, as in recovering precious cargo from a sunken ship. At worst, it means making the best of a bad situation. If prostate cancer comes back the prospect of further destruction is great, and the stakes are high, so the sooner it is detected, the more likely that salvage will "recover" the treasure of life. Send in the reinforcements!

Recurrence after radiation poses a double problem. First, the lifetime amount of radiation that can be delivered to pelvic anatomy has a limit, or cap, so re-treatment with radiation is generally considered inadvisable (a few clinical centers around the country are investigating the feasibility of salvage radiation therapy.) Second, urologists agree that if cancer survives radiation it "comes back pissed" since it's made up of more aggressive, dangerous cells. It may quickly spread beyond the gland into advanced disease (metastasis, or spread). It is important to catch it when the PSA is still well under 10, even around 3 or 4 if possible, since the odds are good that it is still localized and therefore amenable to local control.

Until cryotherapy was developed as a potentially curative salvage strategy, urologists had only two options if a biopsy revealed radio-recurrent cancer: salvage radical prostatectomy (local control) or hormone ablation (systemic control).

RP VS. CRYO AS LOCAL SALVAGE TREATMENT

The obvious salvage treatment that a urologic surgeon would consider is salvage radical prostatectomy, the "gold standard." This would mean surgically removing the entire gland, which makes clinical sense if it can be determined that the recurrent cancer has not yet begun to spread. Naturally, the patient must also be a surgical candidate, able to withstand hours under general anesthesia and face a long recovery. Salvage RP is more complex and demanding than primary RP, and patients are usually several years older than they were when they had primary treatment. Following exposure to radiation in any form, the prostate and surrounding structures are gradually damaged in a way that now makes surgical removal more difficult, though not impossible. The gland has generally shrunk in size, and scar tissue may have formed, fusing it to the adjacent bladder, rectum or blood vessels. An experienced surgeon may have the skill to extract the cancerous gland without much collateral damage, but the risks of incontinence, even rectal damage, are significantly greater than with primary RP; erectile dysfunction is virtually universal. Any patient who was *not* a candidate for surgery the first time around is probably *not* a candidate for salvage RP. Even for those whose age and overall health might qualify them, careful consideration must be given to the risks of side effects.

On the other hand, freezing to kill local recurrence is as effective as salvage RP would be, but with much less time under anesthesia, less chance of permanent incontinence, and less time recovering. The expectation of cure is always somewhat lower with salvage treatment than with primary, because aggressive radiation-resistant cancer may already have begun to spread even when diagnostic tests appear to indicate otherwise. However, even with high-risk recurrence, salvage cryo still offers promising hope of cure. At the 2005 American Urologic Association (AUA) Annual Meeting in San Antonio, TX, Dr. Aaron Katz (New York, NY) presented his 10-year experience with salvage cryotherapy. Of the 157 cases he reported on, 73.3% were biochemically disease free at their most recent follow-up, meaning that their PSA was stable. Incontinence was reported at 6.3%[6], rectal fistula was 0%. Overall, disease-specific survival was 10 years, meaning if patients died during the study period it was due to other causes than prostate cancer. This is comparable to salvage RP survival, but the rate of side effects was appreciably lower than with RP. In fact, at the previous year's AUA Annual Meeting in San Francisco, Dr. Katz debated Dr. Peter Scardino (New York, NY) who argued in favor of salvage RP. Here is a comparison of their reported side effects[7]:

	Salvage Cryo (139 patients) Dr. Katz	Salvage RP (100 patients) Dr. Scardino
Avg. Patient Profile Age PSA Gleason	73.1 12.2 7+	65 10.5 7+
Results Incontinence Rectal injury	2.3% 0%	33% 7%

Notice that the average age of Dr. Katz' patients is older, since cryo can be used with patients who are beyond the age or health limitations for RP, just as with primary cryo. Thus, salvage cryotherapy is my treatment of choice over salvage RP.

Many urologists are still of the mindset that cryotherapy is "experimental" or have not seen the latest data on the low rate of side effects, even for salvage. Such urologists mistakenly believe they have no other choice than surgery for local control of radiation recurrence. If they feel the patient is not a good candidate for surgery, they will automatically turn to the temporary strategy of hormone ablation therapy for temporary systemic control of the disease progression.

HORMONE ABLATION THERAPY (SYSTEMIC SALVAGE) VS. CRYO (LOCAL SALVAGE)

The standard systemic approach to putting the brakes on radiation-recurrent prostate cancer is hormone ablation, often called hormone therapy. It is also the standard of care for prostate cancer that has advanced beyond the gland at the time of diagnosis, or that escaped RP. It is sometimes called "hormone therapy" but the doctor doesn't actually give you hormones. He/she prescribes medication to shut off the pipeline of testosterone to the tumor cells. Prostate cancer is fueled by this hormone, which is mostly produced by the testicles, along with small production from the adrenal gland. Testosterone acts like a "vitamin" to keep prostate cancer vigorous. Therefore, if the tumor cells are deprived of testosterone, they suffer a temporary setback.

Before the advent of salvage cryo, urologists faced with radio-recurrent prostate cancer had no choice but to put non-surgical candidates on hormone ablation therapy as a way to halt the progression of the cancer, especially since it could no longer be assumed that the patient had a "slow-growing cancer" and could afford "watchful waiting."

The common medications given patients offer two basic defense strategies: either *block production* of testosterone, or *prevent uptake* of testosterone by the cancer cells.

Lupron® and Zoladex® are the most common medications that act to *block production* of testosterone. Side effects include hot flashes, impotence, loss of libido, loss of bone density, water weight gain, and mood swings. These are reversible over time if the medication is stopped. (Surgical castration—orchiectomy, or removal of the testicles—also removes the primary production site of testosterone and may result in similar side effects, but it is permanent.)

Casodex® and Eulexin® (flutamide) are the most common medications that *prevent uptake* of testosterone by the cancer cells. Side effects include breast tenderness or enlargement, stomach distress/diarrhea and liver dysfunction. These are also reversible if the drugs are discontinued when warning signs appear.

Before beginning hormone ablation patients must understand that it buys time but is not a cure. Tumor cells that survive radiation are like a pure strain of unrepentant outlaws. They quickly take advantage of any ambush opportunity. Sooner or later, they figure out how to grow even when the fuel is not present. If we only opt to suppress them, we still allow the possibility that these villainous cells will attain immortality and literally spread like wildfire. Now the brakes are off. This is what's called hormone refractory or hormone independent growth. It is the last stage in the life cycle of prostate cancer cells, and the final options for patients are chemotherapy, participation in experimental clinical trials, and palliation (pain relief).

Another consideration before beginning hormone ablation is the effect it will have on quality of life. While adding months or years of time, many men struggle with the side effects. There is no universal equation of how to balance quantity vs. quality of life. A patient and doctor must have a searching conversation, taking into account medical history, life expectancy, lifestyle, and likely disease progression.

If a radiation patient with a 10-year life expectancy develops localized recurrence, and his urologist gives him a choice between a few years on hormone ablation (and a bleak outlook once the tumor outsmarts the medications) or a potentially curative local treatment, how should he approach decision-making?

A HYPOTHETICAL CASE

Let's imagine a 68-year old patient named Lee who had external beam radiation therapy (EBRT) five years ago and is in otherwise good health. After four years of a stable PSA that reached a nadir (lowest point) of 1.2, routine monitoring revealed a rise to 1.8. Six months later it had almost doubled, to 3.1. Three months later it had just cleared 4.0. With three successive rises in PSA, a biopsy is now warranted. His urologist performs a needle biopsy and diagnoses a Gleason 7 (4 + 3) cancer on the right side of the prostate. He next embarks on a manhunt to find out where else it might be lurking. If it's only in the prostate, that's great news, because ice in the prostate can kill these villains. From the result of Lee's other tests (bone scan, ProstaScint®, MRI, for example) it appears that the cancer has not yet spread. There is still an opportunity to destroy the recurrent tumor. These cells have already proven they can resist radiation, so it's a race against time.

If Lee's urologist is not a cryosurgeon, or has outdated beliefs about cryo, he may entertain the possibility of salvage RP, given Lee's age and medical history. If he discards that option, pretty much the only choice left open is hormone ablation therapy. If Lee doesn't know about cryo, he may already be somewhat pessimistic, even fatalistic. He may think, "I spent over six weeks of my life going for daily radiation treatments, and it didn't work. I didn't want surgery the first time around, and I hear it would be even worse now, if it worked at all. What's the use of looking further? Give me the shots or pills or whatever, and I'll just deal with it."

The sad part is, Lee anticipates an inevitable outcome without even knowing he had an additional option in cryotherapy. In his case, it might be a choice for cure. I get frustrated when I hear stories like Lee's.[8]

My best advice is this: If you are a prostate cancer patient who already had primary radiation therapy (beam, seeds or combination) and your PSA is rising, don't wait till it goes over 4.0. See your urologist as soon as possible to learn what is causing it. It could be a harmless, benign condition. However, if a biopsy reveals recurrence, the sooner you obtain accurate information on the likelihood that it is contained, you owe it to yourself to get evaluated as a candidate for salvage cryoablation. Lethal ice destroys all cells that are caught up in it, so the sooner you put them in the path of cryo, the greater your chances of conquest.

Chapter 5.

WHY YOU?

The biopsy revealed a Gleason grade of 9.5. Dr. Scionti went over each treatment option: chemotherapy with radiation; brachytherapy (radioactive seed implant); and cryotherapy. He gave me the full parameters of all three. He did not feel prostate removal was a good option in my case. I knew I did not want chemo, or nuclear medicine, so I decided to go with cryo because it had no chemo or radiation side effects, and could be done outpatient.
Wally C., Patient

If you are a patient with localized prostate cancer and you are exploring treatment options, you have arrived at the most important point of this book: Why should you consider cryotherapy?

Before I review the case for cryo, I want to emphasize that this book is not a substitute for personal medical advice. Only face-to-face dialogue with your physician can help you clarify your alternatives. He or she is qualified to explain your test results and your treatment options. It is crucial that you have adequate information on all choices. If your doctor has strongly recommended one treatment over another, hopefully he or she has acquainted you with why it is in your best interest, and made it easy for you to understand. I speak for myself and all of my colleagues when I say that we want you to have confidence in us, but unless you ask us about what you don't know or understand, we can't be sure that we have covered all the information that an individual may need or want. When it comes to cryo, if by chance your doctor has ruled it out on the grounds that it is "experimental," feel free to pass along this book, or have your doctor get in touch with me. I would welcome a chance to set the record straight!

Having gotten that off my chest, I now want to highlight the aspects of cryo that make it well worth your consideration.

CRYO KILLS CANCER

The foremost advantage of freezing is how effectively it destroys cancer. As you learned, the processes involved in freezing to lethally cold temperatures and doing a double freeze/thaw cycle are destructive to cancer cells in several ways. Some are mechanical and some are biochemical. Put simply, **ICE KILLS CANCER.** Thanks to today's computer-assisted technology, an experienced cryosurgeon achieves equal or greater success when compared with surgical removal of the prostate, or radiating it inside the body.

Remember: no prostate cancer treatment comes with a 100% guaranteed cure. However, if you agree with me that cancer is demolished for good if it is completely encompassed by lethal ice, and if you agree with my research that freezing offers established success equivalent to other treatments and in some cases better, you should consider cryo.

CRYO IS MINIMALLY INVASIVE

Compared with surgical removal, cryo is a minimally invasive procedure with reduced time under anesthesia, outpatient capability, and rapid recovery time. With the use of ultrasound imaging and temperature monitoring, we can get a precision iceball inside the body where we want it, with no cutting or blood loss. Patients often enjoy a return to normal activity within days, and resumption of more strenuous physical activity such as exercise and lifting in a couple of weeks. Patients often report only swelling and/or bruising in the first few days after cryo, and minimal use of over the counter pain medication, if any. In fact, there are rarely any complaints following treatment except for the use of a catheter to drain the bladder for a week, more or less, before it is removed for normal urination. I tell my patients, "We're going to take a short period out of your life, beat your cancer, get you recovered and then you're going to go on with your life." When I explain cryo to them, they have realistic expectations. They expect that for up to a month after treatment they may have minor urinary symptoms, but then they're going to get better. That's the usual experience, and if the pace of recovery is important to you, you should consider cryo.

CRYO IS NON-NUCLEAR

Medicine often walks a fine line between saving life vs. destroying hostile agents such as bacteria, viruses and cancer. The same things that can harm the body (cutting, burning, freezing, poisoning) can be harnessed for good, to rid the body of disease. There are many exciting advances in nuclear medicine for treating cancer. However, many people really don't like the idea of radiation in their bodies.

For many people who came of age after the development of atomic bombs, there is an innate fear of the unseen, uncontrollable effects of radiation scatter, including the mutation of cells into malignancy. I am a firm believer in the "psychology" of treatment choice. Patients seem to recover better and faster when they believe in their treatment. I also espouse the belief that a patient's emotional network offers intangible healing benefits, so when caregivers are themselves uncomfortable with radiation in the body of their loved one, their support may appear ambivalent.

I also pointed out that when a urologist refers patients to a radiation oncologist for treatment, that person will probably not have long-term involvement with the patient. It will be the original urologist who attends to the follow up.

Cryotherapy gives patients an alternative to radiation. Both freezing and radiation are minimally invasive (external beam is technically non-invasive, while brachytherapy uses the same percutaneous entry route as cryo) but the effects of ice are essentially immediate, with visible and fixed treatment planes. Radiation, on the other hand, does its job over time. It's not possible to "see" the treatment as it's occurring, and there is always some scatter effect that may cause side effects, some of which won't show up for years. Remember, I call this "collateral damage." In fact, a 2005 study reported by the University of Minnesota demonstrated a possible link between prostate radiotherapy and an increased risk of rectal cancer.[9] If the thought of radiation in your body creates mental or emotional discomfort for you or your loved ones, you should consider cryo.

CRYO IS REPEATABLE

One of cryo's strongest advantages is that it doesn't burn any bridges for future treatments, especially cryo itself. If cancer recurs and is localized, cryo can be repeated. This is not generally considered true of radiation.

CRYO IS A SALVAGE TREATMENT

Cryo can be used to treat local recurrence after previous radiation has failed. This is especially important since these types of tumors are often more aggressive than the original tumor, perhaps due to selective survival of cancer cells that radiation did not destroy. Remember: Cryo does not discriminate degrees of aggression due to the physics of cell death by ice.

CRYO OFFERS LOW URINARY RISK

In Chapter 1, I went over male pelvic anatomy to show how all prostate cancer treatments entail a risk, however small, of affecting urinary control. New and improved techniques in radical prostatectomy have resulted in reduced incontinence rates, but it still has a significant risk of leaving a patient with a need to use pads for months, and sometimes for the rest of his life. Radiation may also result in urinary side effects that show up later. Cryo has one of the lowest published risks of short- and long-term urinary side effects such as incontinence or painful urination. Here is how I put it to my patients: "We don't want to shoot a mouse with an elephant gun. If I control your cancer so it doesn't progress, but leave you with a pad or painful urination for the rest of your life, I haven't done you any favors. I want a treatment modality that will give you the least risk of long-term lifestyle complications." If the risk of incontinence concerns you, you should consider cryo.

CRYO AND POTENCY

Prostate cancer patients and their sexual partners are rightly concerned about the risk of impotence associated with treatment. I define impotence as the inability to have a spontaneous erection sufficient for penetration. There are different treatment considerations for sexually active patients with low-risk prostate cancer (PSA <10, Gleason score <7, Stage <T2a) than for those with higher-risk disease.

Because total gland cryoablation is associated with high rates of short-term impotence, anywhere from 80-95% for up to a year following cryo, most sexually active men with low risk prostate cancer lean toward either nerve-sparing surgery, if their age and overall health make them good candidates, or brachytherapy if they can't have or don't want surgery. Both of these treatment options offer good cancer control with upwards of 50% chance of preserving erectile function for patients in this category. On the other hand, in a published study 47% of potent men who had total gland cryo regained sexual function within 1-3 years of treatment.[10] This percentage may be even higher if the use of medication and/or a vacuum erection device is initiated soon after treatment in order to keep erectile tissue healthy. In my experience, this form of penile recovery encourages the return of spontaneous erections sooner than if it is not prescribed.

Should younger men with low-risk tumors consider total gland cryo, with its high rate of short-term impotence after treatment? They might not want to rule it out, especially if their cancer is on only one side of the gland. They may be candidates for "nerve-warming" cryo, a technique that keeps one or both neurovascular bundles from reaching lethal temperatures while the entire gland is frozen. They may be candidates for less than a total gland freeze (sometimes called targeted cryo, focal cryo, nerve-sparing cryo, or hemi-cryo).

Since both of these techniques spare some living prostate tissue, patients must undergo more meticulous and extensive initial diagnosis to be sure they don't have multifocal cancer. In addition they must be motivated for more rigorous monitoring following treatment. Perhaps not surprisingly, an unusually high proportion of men drawn to this approach are physicians and engineers who have educated themselves about the science of cryo and analyzed the benefits. Patients for whom nerve-sparing radical prostatectomy is an option—and even men on watchful waiting—may find these factors worth noting: In two different early "focal freeze" studies (Onik; Bahn[11]) 80% of patients who were already potent and underwent a partial freeze were immediately potent after treatment. All were fully continent.

All patients thus treated participate in regular PSA monitoring. Should it begin to rise and localized cancer is found by biopsy, <u>all</u> treatment options—repeat cryo, surgical removal, radiation—are still open. While still being tracked, in some cases the data goes back 6-8 years, and reveals over 90% success in controlling cancer (no recurrence).

If you are sexually active and your urologists say you are qualified for a nerve-sparing radical prostatectomy, you should consider targeted, or "focal," cryotherapy.

OUTPATIENT TREATMENT

Cryo can safely be done on an outpatient basis, allowing you to have your procedure in the outpatient surgery department and sleep in your own bed at night. Prostate cryotherapy is less costly than either surgery or radiation, and results in lower out-of-pocket expenses for patients, and less stress on the economic system. This is especially true in salvage cryo, or cryoablation for recurrence after radiation failure. Before salvage cryo was available, such patients were usually put on hormone therapy, which is expensive, non-curative, and for many men severely impacts their quality of life (see Chapter 4).

In other words, cryotherapy means a same-day, in-and-out treatment, or at most a one-night stay in the hospital when indicated. Patients quickly find themselves back home with a manageable recovery protocol, and an early return to normal activity.

STATE OF THE ART THERAPY

Today's cryo takes advantage of sophisticated technology that integrates imaging, computerized logarithms, physics and biology into a single system, pictured below:

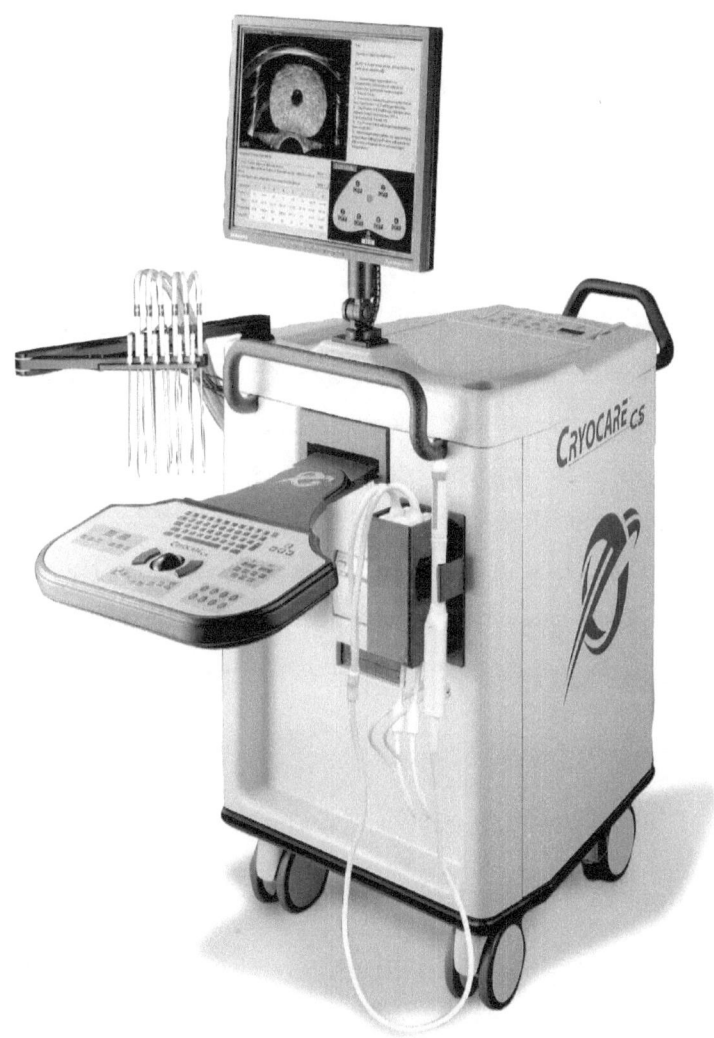

The physician brings surgical training and knowledge to his/her interface with the equipment. This harmony results in a simple formula:
Physician Experience + Technology = Treatment Excellence

Urology as a field has always embraced advances in technical science and engineering, moving toward increasingly patient-friendly treatments of the personal "plumbing" that makes up the genito-urinary system. Witness the adoption of "scope" technology, including laparoscopic radical prostatectomy—even the use of robotics! More than 500 U.S. urologists now perform cryotherapy, and the number is growing. We are rewarded by the high success, rapid recovery, and patient satisfaction we see.

Many of my prostate cancer patients do an Internet search before they make a treatment decision. As fast as up-to-date information is generated, it appears on the Web. Patients can confirm for themselves that the latest developments in cryoablation are far beyond what existed 10 years ago with increasing success rates. They feel confident that freezing offers quick and thorough cancer death with very low risk of side effects.

Cryotherapy has demonstrated great urologic advantages in curing thousands of cases of prostate and kidney cancers. There are now clinical trials testing the feasibility and success of cryo for

- Liver cancer

- Lung cancer

- Breast tumors (benign and malignant)

- Bone cancer (to alleviate pain)

- Cardiac applications (heart arrhythmia, or irregular heartbeat)

If you are convinced that advanced engineering improves medical treatment, you should consider cryo.

CRYO AND IMMUNOTHERAPY

A cardinal principal that guides medical practice is, "Above all, do no harm." The human body tolerates freezing very well. Even the idea of freezing is more acceptable than thoughts of cutting, burning, melting, radiating, poisoning—all of which sound quite aggressive when compared to freezing. In fact, some treatments such as radiation and chemotherapy can adversely affect a patient's immune system while undergoing treatment, a side affect that needs to be attended to so the costs of treatment don't outweigh the benefits. "Above all, do no harm."

Not only does the body seem to accept ice without additional harm—remember those Omaha Steaks and frozen sperm—there is research evidence that in some instances, cryo appears to mobilize the immune system, enabling it to weaken or kill any cancer cells that have begun to spread from the primary tumor. A clinical trial is ongoing to see if these sporadically observed immune responses can actually be pre-programmed to occur using a patient's own dendritic cells in conjunction with tumor cryoablation. It is too soon to say whether this approach, as with other research approaches to a cancer "vaccine," will bear out. However, it is positive testimony that at a minimum, cryo not only avoids unwanted harm, but may even boost the body's own defenses.

LET'S RECAP

You should consider cryo because it

1. Kills cancer.

2. Is minimally invasive.

3. Is non-nuclear.

4. Is repeatable.

5. Is a "salvage" treatment for localized radiation failure.

6. Has low risk of incontinence.

7. Can reduce the risk of impotence for qualified patients.

8. Can be done outpatient.

9. Is state-of-the-art technology.

10. Does no additional harm.

11. May interact positively with the immune system.

I owe so much of who I am and what I've learned to many people who have cared for me and helped me, first and foremost my family. Throughout my life I have also found inspiring teachers and mentors. When I was a urology resident, our program chair was Myron Walzak, M.D. He referred to us as "his boys" and he was like our dad. From an intellectual standpoint, he was one of the greatest influences in my professional career. He was so committed to our education and our success, and he was hard on us but not in a condescending way. He insisted that we ask the right questions. "There is no substitute for information," he would say. "So many times, doctors make an improper diagnosis or prescribe an improper treatment because they don't have all the information." I have his picture in my office, a gentle reminder of how important it is to have sufficient and correct knowledge before making a decision.

I have given you a lot of information about cryotherapy. I hope that by now you are as convinced of its merits as I am. This book is not a substitute for personal care and advice from your own urologist. There is no one treatment that is right for everyone, including cryo. It is not the only treatment I offer, but it's the one many of my new patients are least familiar with and it deserves the fair shake I have tried to give it here. I have explained the aspects of cryo that make it a good choice, perhaps even the best choice, for you to consider. Whatever you do, don't rule out cryotherapy just because someone tells you that it's experimental or results in rectal damage or any other myth that might be floating around out there. Ask yourself if the idea of cryotherapy appeals to you, and discuss it with your urologist.

If you or your doctor has questions about whether you are a candidate for cryo, I would welcome a personal conversation with you or him/her. I can be reached at Coastal Carolina Urology Group, LLC on Hilton Head Island, SC, 1-866-422-2284. You can also reach me through my Cryocare Center website, www.cryocarecenter.com.

But don't just take my word for it. You can see that I am biased in favor of cryo, but I'm not alone. For more information on cryotherapy, visit www.prostatecancer.com.

Whatever you decide, I wish you a speedy and complete recovery if you or a loved one has been diagnosed with prostate cancer.

Note To The Reader: This book is not medical advice, nor intended to substitute for such. It is not the author's intent to give medical advice contrary to that of an attending physician. For questions of a personal medical nature, please consult your physician.

ENDNOTES

* To be consistent with scientific literature I will be using the Celsius scale rather than the Fahrenheit scale. Water freezes at 0° C (Celsius) which is the same as 32° F.

[1] B.J. Donnelly et al. "Prospective trial of cryosurgical ablation of the prostate: five-year results. <u>Urology</u> (Vol. 60, No. 4) pp. 645-49.

[2] Patient's name changed to protect anonymity. Used with patient's permission.

[3] B.J. Donnelly et al. Ibid.

[4] Bahn et al, reported in 2002 in the <u>Urology</u> supplement (Vol. 60, No. 2A) pp. 3-11

[5] Robinson, John W. et al. Reprints of study available through Dr. Robinson, Tom Baker Cancer Center, 1331-29 St. N.W., Calgary, Alberta, Canada, T2N 4N2.

[6] This study goes back 10 years and includes cases done without today's more sophisticated technology. Recent incontinence rates for salvage cryo are as low as 2.3%.

[7] *Cryocare News*, Aug. 2004 (Vol. I, No. 1)

8   It is beyond the scope of this book, but many physicians are aware of the economic savings of salvage cryo, as well as its ability to prolong life and preserve quality of life. If you are curious about how the costs of hormone ablation add up, visit http://caonline.amcancersoc.org/cgi/content/full/52/3/154.

9   http://www.cancer.umn.edu/page/news/release033105.html. Press release issued by UMN, Apr 1 2005.

10 Donnelly, ibid.

11 Onik et al. Dec 07 J Urol 70(6) S1:16-21; Bahn et al. Sep 06 J Endourol 20(9):688-692.